Praise for ANTIBODY

"Elane Kim's exquisite debut makes me think of Gaston Bachelard's thought that 'one must live to build one's house, and not build one's house to live in.' Kim's poems are intricate architectures that refuse to flinch in the face of grief, trauma, and loss with each poem 'searching for sweetness / where there is only dust.' Using a fierce and measured voice, Kim builds a timeless structure that stands firmly against the chaotic forces of the outside world." —ADAM CLAY, author of *Circle Back*

"In *Antibody*, Elane Kim transforms the body into archive, altar, and experiment, writing as both witness and scientist, daughter and maker. These poems are ablaze with hunger, precision, and tenderness, carrying us from kitchen smoke to hospital rooms, from Gyeongju's dust to California drought, from the dream of a homeland to the ache of its distance. Kim's gift is her ability to hold contradiction without collapsing it: the poems live in both wound and wonder, grief and astonishment. 'Sometimes, the only thing separating a body from grief is more grief,' she writes, and the book follows that logic, turning loss into a language that sings. The lyric is deeply sensorial—full of cicadas, moon jars, soft pears, ginseng, soot—but also electric with scientific clarity: 'I paint / entire lineages radioactive green, / stained fluorescent with protein.' This is a collection preoccupied with survival—but survival, here, is not flat endurance but radiant invention. Kim interrogates what it means to be daughter, immigrant, citizen, poet, to inherit not just language but silence, hunger, and the histories of others. She makes of those inheritances something startling and new—sonnets that teach the body to speak, diptychs that reimagine myth, manifestos that reassemble language syllable by syllable. At its heart is the insistence that nothing—not grief, not estrangement, not exile—is beyond re-making. This book is an act of devotion, an offering of light."

—KIMBERLY GREY, author of *Systems for the Future of Feeling*

"'Everything we love does not belong to us.' Elane Kim's *Antibody* is a sweeping and elegiac book about grief and language and vision. It's about what can be seen through, and in, the dying light. It's a book written by a formally restless and inventive poet torn between two languages and two traditions, trying to find a home. What do you do when you can't find a home? You have to create one for yourself. *Antibody* is that creation."

—JOSH BELL, author of *The Gods in Small Doses*

ANTIBODY

ANTI

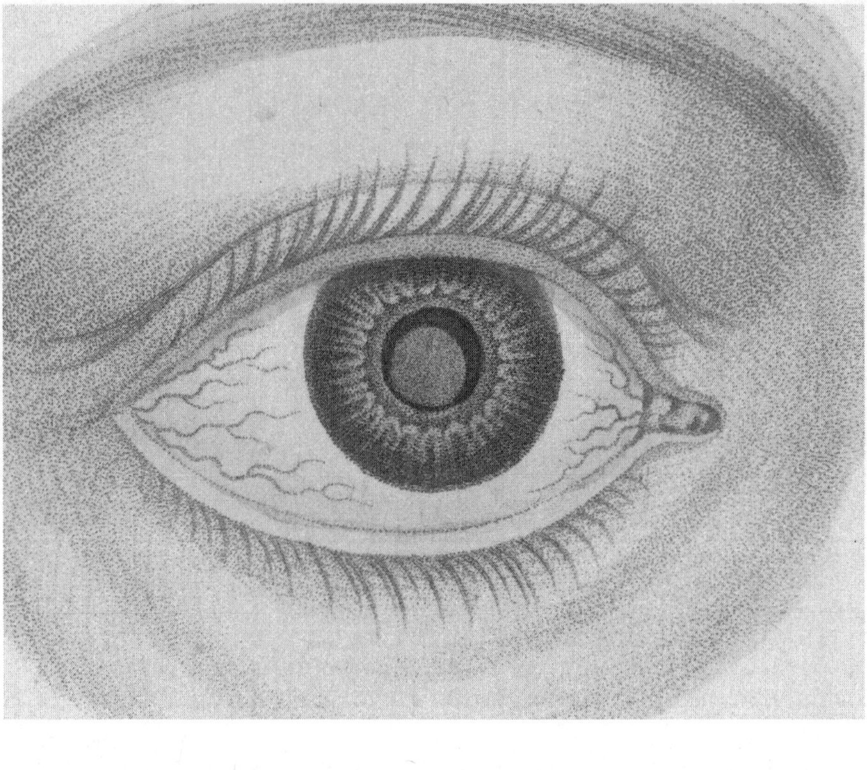

ELAN

BODY

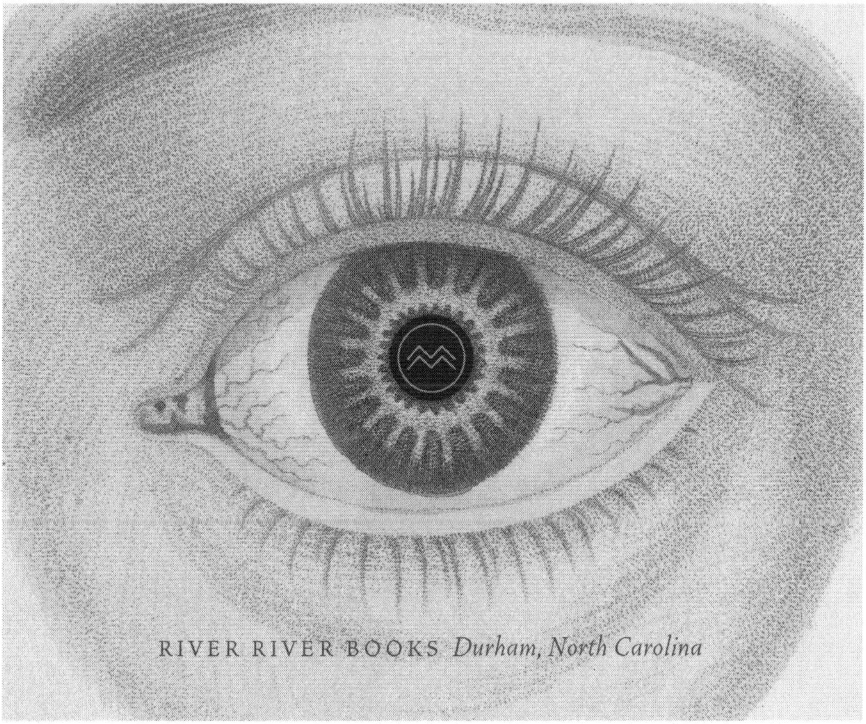

RIVER RIVER BOOKS *Durham, North Carolina*

E KIM

Published in the United States of America

Library of Congress Cataloging-in-Publication Data
Kim, Elane, 2004–
Antibody / Elane Kim.
ISBN-13: 979-8-9926116-0-1
Subjects: LCSH: American Poetry,
Asian-American Poetry, Science, Medicine, Grief
LCGFT: Poetry.
LCCN: 2025942190

Cover and interior design by Alban Fischer

RIVER RIVER BOOKS
10 Linganore Place
Durham, NC 27707

www.riverriverbooks.org

For my dear family

CONTENTS

I. BRIGHT-FIELD

"I am the immigrant clutching the hope I seek—"

—Langston Hughes

SUITE D

I want to be the discount bookstore and all its stock, the copper bell
at its door. I want to be bright scarves, soft rain, seabirds
pecking at receipts. I want to be the stripe of pepper
on your cutting board, the expensive cut at the supermarket. Its film

of fat and the way it sticks to you. I want to be honest. I swear.
I can only say what I mean. I mean my face is your face. My country is your
country. I want this to be true, to be hydrogen peroxide:
the hiss, the foam at your mouth. To be like rain,

an open wound. The floodgates after the first bite. There are jungles ripe
with this kind of wildness. The sky, pale-orange, is only a measure
of the asbestos in our lungs. I want you to hold yourself
like an armful of birds. Not a bullet or a burning field or just

a body. I believe in so much that isn't there: a soft apple
bruised and alive, wildfires leaking in the backyard, a pulse
as you sleep. Give me something I can outlast. Give me more
to call my own. An apron, an old encyclopedia. The dying streetlights

or a beehive in front of the brown vitamin store. There is shelter
to the smoke somewhere, enough square feet of granite, enough time
to pay the rent. Survival doesn't have to be an act
of loneliness. I promise I will say grace. I will be your wheatgrass,

yes. The way it sticks to you. Photographic film, expired film, overripe
fruit. The ceramic bowls you never use for yourself. Your red packets
of ginseng extract, raw peanuts, a whole hometown of bitterness.
A poem to fit in your mouth.

SECOND TRY

Distance is an excuse for estimation. Home is
a repetition of sounds, the ones that know
how to burrow: metal pots and metal birds,
sharp rain and the squeal of rubber. Absolute value:
language measured by its displacement, its echo,
its distance from home. So long as it's something
I can repeat. Something I can get wrong the first try
and love by the second. I find warmth for the first time
many times. Once in the gauze of the care unit.
In the restaurant booth and again at table four.
Once despite your hands. Once despite mine.
When there were birds and only birds,
we stopped resenting our wingless bodies. By now,
I can be sure: the summer I am still so afraid
is the summer I am less honest. It's loud
and now the birds are all gone. I don't remember
all your pieces. Only the way they slotted
into place.

TRANSCRIPTION, PHONE CALL, APRIL

for Halmeoni / for Eomma

Birds have their homing instinct.
Despite migration, magnetic forces.
A mother's voice telling you to stay.
Do you know 사철나무?
These blue blue trees that tower like men.
How every day your Halmeoni would speak to them like children.
잘커라, she would say.
Grow well, to you trees who know nothing else.
But they never grew taller, only stubbier, heads wiry and glaucous.
So Halmeoni spoke with the deer, this family of deer who had eaten the boughs and the hairs and the lips of every branch in secret.
Who said nothing.
Their green eyes starving and gorgeous.
So Halmeoni began to hate the deer which she had once cherished, or at least said as much.
I think she was lying.
She was a girlish soul, your Halmeoni.
Like the bluest tree.
She loved to dance.
Can't you write something about this?
She was a girl, the way she fluttered like blossoming birds, shining even when unpolished.
You know how blue and green sound the same in our language.

Our language that never cries.
Tell me you will call more often.

BILDUNGSROMAN

Desires, according to Calvino, are already
memories. This is a way of saying that
language is a fist of snakes, that it is too late

for remorse if you are watching
another invisible city burn. My throat
is a thing of contradiction: too many

unoiled syllables collecting into sharpness.
The autumn of my birth,
my mother tells me, *You must know this—*

your name means harvest. And so
another generation is raised on quiet prayer,
heads bowed, drinking spools of smoke

and river water. Desires, according to my mother,
are best left unspoken, unopened. And yet
she cracks open the back of a snow crab, splits

its bright body into shards, leaves
the redness on my plate. This is a way of saying
there is no way to know which body is yours,

whose home is burning. Desires, according to nobody
in particular, are gray, finicky things,
things to be worn and then returned.

In the same way, I imagine my mother's past self—
the quiet line of her mouth, the softness
of her lies. My name has always meant drought.

PRE-FLOOD DIPTYCH

I.

Slow rise of the morning like
insides brewing, swirled into paste.
A moon jar holds nothing but exile, distortion,

a lifetime of war spilled like water.

Harabeoji's body locked inside
the whitest room of a shrinking palace.

Ailing body. White as
the scratch of our old stucco walls.
The zenith of Eomma's stomach, hanging

like a moon, still heavy with life.

II.

It was a happening place, scene
loose with water
and the compound eyes of cicadas.

The moor blackened,
ruined by rain.

Everyone watching at once
to see who would drown
before our futureless language.

Before the child could even breathe,
he was buried.

Now I want every rain to feel
like the first. I want fruit like you wouldn't
believe. Skin bruised by light, body

dense as flesh, atomically radiant.
I swallow the lukewarm glass and
shed my eyes.

There is no time.

No future tenses.
Only the distance to white
poplars, their nesting sparrows.

Only the long walk home.

DEAR READER

Lately, the weather has been kind. One stop
away from Central, the snow is rare and pale. It glitters like
it's the last time you'll ever see it.   You know how it feels

to be blanketed in fluorescence and geysers of salt. To want nothing
more than to return home wrapped in a family. Because
our cells are soft, confer softness, and because

our blood always knows to trickle in the right direction,
towards breath. The weather is   kind. The day is new.
Time is measured in light and so are our bodies and

do you really never die in your dreams? The rest of the day
I'll be waiting. Like someone hailing a yellow cab
or asleep in a hospital. Waiting for life   to arrive.

AXIOM

The most fundamental facts of the universe must be taken as true,
or else nothing will make sense. The fact is that I am trying to be
honest. I can't hold a note for more than twenty seconds.
There are words in Korean with no English equivalent
whose shapes I trace and study. Translation is an act
of replacement. Eomma's words becoming my
apologies. So I believe in unobservables, action
at a distance, fluorescent green rain boots. I believe
the weather forecast and then the diagnosis.
Did you eat today? Which way did your pillow
face? Can you stomach *juk*? Which nurse came
to see you? Are there many birds outside the window?
Were you always so quiet? I believe in so much
that isn't there: a wildfire, a box holding your face,
embroidered in red, apples and tangerines, burning
bodies, bowls scraped clean. Despite your body, you are
here. Nothing makes sense. The loneliest parts of the world
are still trying to be found. I want there to be warmth, even if
it cannot be mine. Will you eat tomorrow? What lies north
of the pillowcase? Can you stomach the uncertainty of rain,
microwaved porridge, the open door? Do you have something left
to say? What are you watching, if not the birds?
Are you already gone?

COROLLARY

There are many ways to be born, though
I have forgotten most. Between miles and miles of orange land:
bellflower root, perilla leaf, mugwort, stigma. In a trainwreck,
a locked bathroom, a pool hall, a village thatched with fire. After rain
as it falls in hot sheets. Before rinsing the bones soft. There is room
for the terrible summer and all its alleyways, too. For quiet. For grief.
I want to follow the fragile light, to find its beating pulse
beneath the floorboards. So many small disasters
to call our own, these calamities we call bodies. Stars
so dim and round I mistake them for eyes. I blink
and I am on a moving train, a sink yellowed with grease.
Birthrights I carry in my sleep. For sorrow. For sickness.
For richer or poorer. For the poplar trees, the pink light weaved
into church windows. I want another armful of flowers. Not fields
of weaponry. The night of the memorial service, caterpillars bloom
in the black of the yard. It's as if it's day. As if it's morning
and there's something alive underneath it all,
patient. Taking watch,
keeping face.

MIDWINTER

And all I want is a warmer month. Mayflies and an open window. The cold without its cruelty. All I want is to stop embodying disaster. To be the moment before impact when everything was still breathing, still making do. A kind of volcanism friendly to salvation. 하느님. I don't want to be bitter. I want to love   love. I want a word for this feeling. The chemical symmetry of our bodies. I am the sum of my parts, or I want to be. Two consenting particles. Impossible people imbued with impossible light. But there is no possibility of replacement, only cartilage torn all the way down. It is so hard not to be swallowed by this great white   whale of a feeling. This crystalline light, organ-like in its beating. The way the linen catches it. This awareness of every body, every countryside and its uncountable remedies for heartbreak. So far from home it feels near-infinite.

SONNET AS FIRST WORDS

Say *ah.* Say *eomma*. Say *appa*. Say, aren't you too old
to be learning English? Say *apple*. Say *appel*. Say
there is more to the world than where your knees
have kissed the pavement. Say *spit*. Say *sorry*. Repeat after me:
native speaker. Say grace. Say, *This is my home*. Let's say
you love her, and she doesn't love you back. Call it language.
Don't you know the present tense of *wound* is still *wound*?
Say *mother*. Say *father*. Say it over again. Let your tongue
become a washboard, your body past tense, your body minor
chord. Say *amendment, contraction*, the declaration
like a prayer. Say *warzone*. Say *warzone*. Say,
I am waiting for this country to love me back. Future
tense. Repeat after me. Stay quiet. Stay quiet. Stay
a little longer. Say *eomma, appa*.

GOOD DAUGHTER

Based on the Korean myth of "Princess Bari"

This is a story   about
birth,   the act of slipping into rivers
and bad luck streaming into daughterhood. A way of   drowning
when there is   no water, only miles   of open field, a wired forest, puffs of

death
hidden behind   camphor   trees. The carp   floating in the sky
so loose-tongued and clever, streaming in the wrong direction. The stork heavy
with clouds. The road to harvest cannot be followed, only   discarded. There is an

open door
and sometimes an open   mouth and always
too many caskets to keep   holding onto. Bari, youngest   daughter, seventh
-born. Girl plunged   into death for a bloodline that

does not love her
back. O   love. O loving. Bari,   meaning good   girl,
bright girl, filial girl,   meaning
there is   some place that will love her best

when she is gone.

This is a story   about
misfortune. Daughter born fish
-tailed, scaled, oceanless. No   ending: only miles
of forest, a place so   green   it could burn   you. Look around:

that square of earth
is somebody   else's. That star is not yours,
never yours. Daughter discarded,   born
        to die, ready to speak   to the dead. So many rivers of yellow blood,
    steaming bile,

enough to drink
a body from. And   when even
this body is not enough   to silence the dead, there will be
nothing left   to grieve. Dear God, dear   grief. Seventh daughter Bari.

Bari,
meaning *to throw   away*,   meaning
wordless   thing, meaning
no good,   meaning

girl.

This is a story about
absence. Girl born   not
son, fish   -mouthed, slick with the blood of another
saint. Too clever   for her own good, too loud   to speak to

the dead.
Too many rounded corners, mouth open   to catch
sharp rain   like bullets. A tailed daughter means   no good,
means severed bloodlines and childless coffins.

This is a story about
cruelty.   Fingers ready to slice
the sky   open, face still mouthless, gaping, breathless.
O Bari, you shivering thing, you   dead thing.   Look around:

all this,
even that bright sun, belongs to you. So let us be   loose-tongued
and clever. Let us love   what makes us   no good
girls, griefless   girls. Let us have

ourselves
this open field and this terrible   body
and a burning match and licks of bitter
kerosene and

still no water.

PROSPECT THEORY

Walnut Creek, 2014

We are good for the first few years. We buy string-knit gloves,
hose attachments. We mind the sun and the cicadas,
the morning weather forecast. *Bad dirt*, Eomma says.
This is not Gyeongju, a city ripe with heat, skewered with smog,
melting still. This is why we lose hope
in the lemon tree so quickly, bury what's left
in our stomachs. Six years for one Meyer lemon
is a terrible investment, if nothing else. I consider
its membrane separating country from country, the way
the roots of the lemon tree float above their shallow grave.
Eomma buys backup seeds: lilac, lavender, catmint.
We stop being so diligent, so kind. We lose hope
in all things displaced, replanted, watered every
other Wednesday. When the first lemon sprouts,
Eomma twists her mouth into a flower: lilac, lavender,
catmint. We know lemon skins grow gray with time. Ours will
lose its sour prick of scent, its brightness. Still, we press it
into a page of paper, thin enough to bleed through. Still, we hang it
over the mantel, hold it to our chests.

WHEN I SAY I AM HUNGRY

I am talking about the immediacy of family: dishes stacked tall,
soot slipping through our hair like rain.

We speak thorns. We swallow paper. We watch stars precess,
bodies ready to explode. I forget the heat, the cold, a little

while longer until closing time. I forget your wrists
littered with grease burns, cool ointment rubbed off

in the heat. Evening raw like something you chew and spit out.
Tobacco blooms on concrete, the stir of your hands reaching

for a jagged mop, for survival. We say smoke. We eat skies. Eat
our fill of summer and then some. Children stop to watch the sky.

You never look up from the cutting board. I want a day without
burning. No more aprons drenched dark in saltwater

brine. Stomachs gurgling like beer. Fat and oil sucked into flesh.
We stay quiet. We stomach emptiness, eat sluggishly: fish bones

and soft-skinned pears, the teeth of an animal and a side of salad.
Just a little music to wash out the rain. You, fluorescent light swiped

against your skin, a picture of a rusted city, its highways tolled,
someplace we can't afford to love. You teach me long division

on old receipts. You make me sit straight. And even when
there are no empty booths, when your insides are raw, bruised like fruit,

even then, you feed me first: a stretch of dough, steaming hot. Something
I can burrow into like sleep. I talk sweet. I drink soft.

I am so hungry,
so full.

II. STRAY LIGHT

"I have a disease: I see language."
—*Roland Barthes*

HOST CELL

After 기형도

and can this body be a prayer if not a home
                                                                  a humming garden if not a prayer   soft
-organed if not a garden
                                                                  like seoul in its leanest years and ribless still
can it be clean as metal, sloe-eyed, vision
unclouded by mugwort   beetroot   tender chrysanthemum
fernbrake or bracken fiddleheads, bitter death
                                                                  we swallow despite

                                                                  can this body be a home

TRANSIT

I want more small kindnesses:
glass stained in every direction,
the windows stacked tall,

a looping stop. Pick a side already: the sky

or the sea. More rain or bullets
still soft with skin. The open river
or the open door. Your blood or mine.

Transpose your life onto a railway track

and see if you can make it home
with one ticket. Memorize the timetables.
I want to point in any direction

and say *I love so-and-so* and mean it.

Love like shades of snow against dirt. Love like
soft hands, blue tongues, tangerine peels
painted over in gesso. Like warmth framed

and stuck on the ceiling fan, or

so many birds on the ocean floor.
I must have missed my stop. Play a song
before you go.

POST-OPERATIVE CARE

"Each evening we are poorer by one day." —*Arthur Schopenhauer*

What is remedy?

The season of prayer that lasted a lifetime.

What is remedy?

Bodies painted bone white and the bluest blue. Colors defying light.

What is remedy?

The act of fisting canopies of light. Rinsing your stomachs of hunger, your bodies of foreign objects. Rinsing yourself clean.

What is remedy?

A body soft with moss, torn with disaster, raw like fever, its unforgiving light. Remembering that you are made of so much hunger and not enough bite. Everything you love is meant to be swallowed.

What is remedy?

We take a walk by the riverside, the first place you think of after the appointment. We eat sweet sunlight and marvel at butterflies and sit with our grief. The butterflies are small and live accordingly. You are small and wingless. We laugh at how our cells come with instructions that they choose not to follow. You, deterministic and still unsure about whether you will wake to see tomorrow. I wonder when you outgrew your body. When the butterflies stopped singing or when you will come home. The last month we shared, the sunlight was not sweet, but it was good and fresh, acidic in its ferocity. I think I am still carrying it with me.

What is remedy?

Everything except for our bodies, your skin mutated into memory. Ecological succession and flowers stained with dew. Gallons of saltwater brine against the methane blue of your lips, my unfaithful tongue, bluest blue, reddest red. Everything you never got to see.

What is remedy?

Skin petrified into flakes, fragile as snowmelt.

What is remedy?

Heads bowed in the most patient act of love I know.

What is remedy?

A way to cling to the ruin. To make it last.

SONNET AT THE SUPERMARKET

His eyes wash over families of fruit, crushed cardboard, sticky
hands. The trick is to be molecular and precise: a watermelon sick
with jaundice is no good, mushy on the inside. Carries disease
internal to itself. Like how cells hold instructions for their own
death or how birds always know the way home. His eyes washed
with chemical droplets and still unseeing. Like light flushed
down the sink. A shade of white so brutal it could kill you.
You have to choose the roundest, brightest fruit, says Appa.
Glaucoma, from *glausso*, from *glow*, the consequences of a blurred
closeness, of seeing beyond yourself. Any wound but this.
The fruit with the darkest stripes. It is a kind of science. Like
the weather forecast and like poetry. His eyes wash over
his daughter's face. The bravery of searching for sweetness
where there is only dust.

1967

경주 — city with air that sticks
    silhouette stamped right on my throat
skin slick with soot   dry with dust   choked with cicada
song
    summer in the brightest years
    winter when the sun dries   red red   government officials
        and their red red   grins

    경주 — city of hunger   of teeth of martyr
    after martyr after martyr after war after war
        after

        what comes after   war

    so I have watched the swallowing
    without a mouth of my own
    so this is how it ends
경주 — glimmering city   drowned city   city
        whose people are hungrier than they are
        alive

NORTH STAR

Zeno's paradoxes of motion: pluralities have no place in the world of the
living.   This is why I learn   and unlearn   my maiden name. I bury
what can fit   in ten square feet: the canned rain, the river. I commit   to
tragedy, the lesser of two evils.   The shallows   of the city   are meant to
be drowned in.   Believe it.   I ask the neighbors if they've seen a bursting
moon, the North Star,   all the pieces of

light we string together   and hang on the mantle.   At night, I dream
of rust and rain   and other quiet pleasures.   I ask my body   what it
means to survive   in a language   punctuated by blank   space   and
it laughs.   The radio swallows the rest   of the anthem.   I sleep for a
while,   long   enough for light to collect   in white cones.   Hidden
beneath the dirt, hibiscus in small patches: red as a secret,   as shame.
Someone says   collisions are the stuff of universes.   I dodge. I mourn.

There is light in a way that stops feeling bright. O the things
we cultivate in place of self: homes, warm fireplaces, cold prayers, great
bronze statues of dead men, fool's gold, the morning after the new year,
the year after the new body, the first supper, the last meal, children
wrapped in red scarves, red for prayer, red for disaster, red, red, relief,
roofs thatched over with whatever will survive.

GLORIA

"Love is my religion." —*John Keats*

I call you 정 first. This is before
you and your sister fight over the name Eunice,

the color white, the bus ride home. I call
the people I know by their names

and the people I don't by the color of their eyes:
blue, green, blue. I pray on Sundays, wave hello

to the mailman every Monday. You collect nail tacks,
thumb slips of lined paper: *property of America*. I organize

the chewing gum by color, the places by sound.
There is the kitchen with the buzz of its linoleum

floors. There is the yard with its pebbles and their sputter.
There is where we sleep. I stack the magazines

tall by the register. I press all the digits on the landline,
enough for an address, enough for a body.

Your tongue becomes a paperweight
and the linoleum sours under my feet. You have a son,

then a daughter. I stop going to church.
The same scenes roll and lurch on the television screen:

screaming woman, looping laugh track.
Every frame shining in all the wrong ways—

blue, green, blue. I call for home: 정-정-정
-정. I call again. There are ways of forgetting

that don't involve memory. I wave to the mailman.
I let the door click shut behind him.

FIELDNOTES

Based on the traditional Korean folk song "Arirang"

Past Baekdu mountain,
there is more land.

Past the river,
there is more
to live for.

The first thing
a mother teaches
her daughter is that
spines take root
where tongues
end.

Listen to the river,
the way it echoes
like a country

creeping into famine.

Look at the fruit trees,
the crepe myrtle,

the white
of the farmer's fence.

Let persimmon peels
collect skin by skin.

Something inside you
is always blooming,
limbs buckling like agarose,
growth rings curling
into bright strands of rain.

You are only
what is left behind

of summer, everything
that has not
stopped burning,

incomplete
combustion of light.

The last thing
a mother teaches
her daughter
is how to sing
without a mouth.

Look past the mountain,
its rot and its bloom.
Past the mourning river
and the shrinking banks.
Past the yellow-lit city

you failed to inherit.

You have always been
a forest.

MURDER HORNETS

The night I moved out of the old home, Appa turned the air conditioner on for the first time. It made a buzzing noise, a noise like a sad bee, so we laughed. I left Appa a Tupperware container of spaghetti in the fridge. Two minutes in the microwave, I said, and he nodded. He and I lived in a small house where we lived small lives: cereal for breakfast, takeout if we saw Appa's check from the factory before the water bill. Then the housing market got competitive. The houses grew taller, wider, and so did the people. We stayed small, and small was enough. Then Appa stopped getting called to the factory, the weeds grew tall in the front yard, and small was less than enough. The night I left, I taught Appa how to use the dishwasher for the last time. *I know this much*, he said, voice flat and sinking, and I nodded this time. We said our goodbyes: *Remember to call. Eat well. Two minutes in the microwave.* When I had walked thirty feet, I peeked through the window: Appa was hanging over the sink, wiping his plate, holding the Tupperware close to his body. I kept walking. I settled in a new city within a new county and lived a medium-sized life. I called Appa to say hello, to tell him about the blue houses and the blue pigeons, to remind him that nectarines were in season. Sometimes, in the quiet of the rain, I would catalog what I had left behind: milk swirling in pale ceramic bowls, elbows at the table, cicada songs, soft orange wind. In the mornings, I watched the news: market crisis, election results, giant hornet found in our old county for the first time. The reporters called it a murder hornet and played its cry. It was a sad sound, waxy and sinking. Familiar. I laughed, and then I thought of Appa: his crumpled body, his crumpled wings. Then, his voice playing over the phone, cracked and unfamiliar: *You can stay longer, you know. You can stay*

as long as you like.

DUPLEX IN SAN FRANCISCO

After Frank O'Hara

There is home in this body
somewhere, I am sure.
    A home is still a home
    without light, without
a welcome mat at the mouth.
This is something I do not learn
    until the light bulbs
    and prayers expire with a gasp,
until my shadow becomes a
bitter song. Cicadas redden the front
    yard with decay. There is no need
    for windows in an empty house. I eat
buildings and bones. When I say
I am sure, I mean to say I am waiting
    for the weeds to grow back.

BLIND SPOTS

A garden ripens under your skin. Begonias shrieking
red, cut to bloom. I think it's too early for these things.

I hope the gardener forgets his hat at home. I hope there is
soft rain, enough to lose trust in the weather forecast,

and then only drought, parched tongues, the pulsing ache of stars
when there is no one to keep watch. I give you

marigolds and a sprig of myrtle. Stigma
and stamen. You unfurl petal by petal: your hands

thorns, your mouth thorns, your body a soft bed
of moss. Has the rain always felt so sharp?

How long have we been poking ourselves raw
with our own skin? Look. There is time

for the terrible hospital room and its assembly of chattering men.
There is time for our two bodies: locked in

eternal summer, our mouths bright as begonias, bright
as feverish crowd and heat stroke. Reddest red as a shade

of blinding, brutal in its whiteness. Bones pale enough to pass
for prayer. Look up. You are still here. The stars are watching, patient,

and the gardener is waiting at the door and you are still
here and who could mistake the light, dappled in dark spots,

for noise, for open window? Who could mistake the light
for anything but ourselves?

SURVIVAL // FOOTNOTES ON SURVIVAL

Eomma's warm [1] soups. Shiny secrets,
humble and dangerous. [2] The uncertainty [3] principle
in action. Cold leftovers [4] and condensed steam.
Forest fires sprouting in [5] the faraway hometown, or
the sharp wind of cars zipping on the freeway.
Something other than [6] the layers of dust
and water, something beyond it all. A little forest,
bright [7] with fuschia wildflowers and a bed of rolling hills.
Staring at the [8] sun. The trees and
their infinite [9] eyes.

1 Warm light to keep
2 us company. What more could we ask for but
3 certainty in our joy? Our sorrow, too,
4 oversized and bloated. Like tongues.
5 In the absence of music, we
6 thank the people we love and
7 write songs out of our softness. Because
8 the body is a soft place. As soft as it is
9 finite.

SONNET OVERHEARD AT PHONE BOOTH

Goodbye, but said without really meaning it. The way
the light touches you like something scared. Or my armful
of sunspots and the milk expiring on the countertop
and many unopened tubes of paint and hair ties
lost to the unmanicured wild. The sheer loneliness
of your body on the cosmic scale. There's so much
I'm not telling you: orange tickets, limpid rain,
the last train home. The kindness of every shadow, the way
something patient keeps count beneath the rib cage.
Goodbye, meaning, *I will see you right after this call.*
Meaning, *I am leaving a message at the tone and a song*
that will loop and a bird or two to peck at all the crumbs
I have left behind. Meaning, *I am still here, listening,*
waiting for the train to arrive.

RESPITE

It's New Year's.
It's New Year's and the stars are white-hot and all your favorite dishes
are flushed warm on the island: ddeok-guk for fortune, knife-cut noodles
for longevity, persimmon pudding and a tin can of sardines.
The nectarines are in season in our backyard and the pigeons
are painting their pale bodies with rain. The man in the powdered apron
still feeds them on the porch of his square little store, the way you said
was too generous. Too much for such small bodies to be eclipsed
by hunger. We leave flowers by your pillow, the lakeside whirring
with cicadas. We chose a round pound cake from the supermarket
last week, the anniversary of your funeral. I confuse my birthday
with the day you died. Are you listening? I am still making a list
of places for us to visit: the static image of your youth,
the last lake in which you loved. There should have been
more distractions. There are still so many sardines
left in their cans, floating belly-up in brine. Seabirds still float
against the red bridge, arrogant, flashing their bellies
toward the sky. I think you would have liked to feed them.
I think you would have been generous,
despite.

III. AFTERIMAGE

"She says to herself if she were able to write she could continue to live."

—*Theresa Hak Kyung Cha*

EATING KIMCHI ALONE

For Appa

Our bodies are so full of potential space and the world
is mostly empty. It is a contradictory biology: scalars and teeth, blood
and soft water. Paradise, California, and it all erupts into flames. So
the daughter never grows into herself. So I was blastula until I divided,
amniotic and split at the mouth, a creature impossibly alive. Bilateral like pea flowers
or fish gasping for air or the Rorschach in which I saw a laughing father
instead of a butterfly. Appa wants me to write a poem about eating kimchi alone
in San Francisco. Dinner for one in the large, pale dark. Hunger tempered
by the smell of ammonia. There is a difference between loneliness and solitude
that I am still looking for. Maybe I am always lonely, even when
I am laughing, especially when I am laughing. I want to name a city after this feeling.
I want a body calculus-smooth, suspended in amber, totally unconcerned
with what comes after it. No more fake heavens that shine like eyes. No more
teeth. Odd function, evaluate to zero, convince myself that the data are not ugly,
just crunchy with noise. So much of this world is empty space, meaning
we are half of it. The kimchi ripens, so I promise myself laughter.
So I write the poem. So I bite. Like formaldehyde or a hometown, it floods,
then burns. It's a quiet love, this dinner for one. It's unending. We live
in it.

SIGHTLINES

After the diagnosis
I dream of sugar and soft things to chew on.
I dream of seeing you as you were—eyes
not glaucous, not blooming. You light
-shaped thing. You daughterless thing.
Invisible cities, Calvino says, are not homes.
Not because they are invisible but because
we are blind. And so I dream about whales blessed
with both movement and sight. Our bodies with half
the blubber and half the flight. Last summer fragmented
into wet cherries and wetter clothes. Because every day
is a new day in America. America, where the sun rises
in the east and the city always contains you. Contains.
Containing still. Candles grow bright with prayer,
then wane into memory. Everything borrowed
and nothing yours. So here is evidence of flowing water:
a conglomerate of unseeing green, this catastrophic flood
that never left my mouth. The night of the surgery,
I dream I give you a bouquet of violins
strung by their noise, their violent thrum,
and I wake clutching my chest. Surrounded by green youth,
clean teeth, soft-eyed men walking to urgent
appointments, your arrival many exits from home.
Retina translated from a glacier: skinned

thing, glittering thing, something that shines brightest
just before it's gone. Your eyes red and swollen.
Because the redder the light, the farther you are from it.
Because many planets ago, there was no light.
That's how we enter the world, with our blindness
and our ache. That's how we are born.
That's how you live.

A CHILD IS BORN

a flower that opens once in a lifetime.

Temporary light, pindrop of silence before insurmountable death. A snowdrop
on a hill, surrounded by numbness. He learns the language of aphids
and echoes their silent screams. Always the same story:
boy, snowdrop, forest, so many miles from home.

A child is born the son of a government official and a home-
maker. Eldest son, well-bred and humble. Learns poetry, philosophy,
how to paint mountain landscapes and pale horses. When he closes his eyes,
he leaves snowdrops unfinished, dipped in fragile light.

A child is born in a war and wrapped in a second skin.
Quick as instinct, he learns he must tear it off in a big peel. Waxy
and uninhabitable. Like a brother, only smaller, weaker, uglier,
constricting breath, constricting song.

A child is born a faceless land, split at the seams. Learns hunger
in the absence of green. When townsfolk spray noxious pesticides like something
sweet, toxins in great plumes, he and his brother chase the comet tails
of their trucks, mouths open in laughter, shrieks muffled by rain.

A child is born. He is the second son, his appetite endless. He has a son of his own, then a daughter. Dreams of rainstorms or apocalypse. Some world, this world, his to inhabit, soft with firelight and fruit. It is a barren country he pretends is tender. *I could tell you a lifetime*, he tells his languageless daughter.

I could tell you a lifetime.

AUBADE IN THE AFTERMATH

Say there is a time for breathing and a time for stillness. Say
there is no place for mourning. It's easy to know these things.

You can learn to exhale. Let the marrow of dusk leak
onto your knees. We are just soft bones and the places they inhabit.

The act of silence: heavy as rain. Heavy enough to believe in.
We have never been strangers to translation,

the language of crookedness. You find hunger in the health
inspector's mouth, in antiseptic and ginger. I find it in day

-old receipts and papercuts. Tongues rattling, we are scared
into daughters again and again. Our lungs

the shape of drowning. Someone will always want
to dissect your body, peel it wing by wing. There will be

no vaults wide enough to hold it. So I will take it
home with me. I will give it a toothbrush and softness

and one-half of the bed. We can start like this: at noon, with bird bones.
How to continue: tomorrow, with forsythia in fistfuls. Yes,

we have always been strangers to song. This is why
we scatter our hands to the wind again and again. Yes,

hunger is sometimes a symptom of grief. This is why
there are no instructions for healing, no recipe for light. Yes,

forgiveness will come with the slowness of rot. This is why
we are waiting.

MIDSUMMER

Your bed plucked apart, stripped like a bird, and cold dew washing the grime off our teeth. I wake to a moon, dim and yellow, forcing its limbs through the kitchen shutters. Learning to live in this skin without grieving. Learning I am citizen only when I am naked of my voice, its animal croak. Child rounded to the nearest integer. A story invented out of nothing   but want. I can give you hunger or I can give you an unspeakable fullness. The radius of our desires or that of our quiet or just the inevitability of my empty hands. Wipe the table and take the order. Take the order.

The distance pierces, leaves in its wake

a heavy wound, dim and yellow.

SONNET WITH KITCHEN GREASE

The restaurant never closes, only opens, its doors gaping wide like a mouth,
a cavity. Here I learn long division, hyphenation. All the remainders
of things. I name every bird in the elbow of our junction: *nabi*, then *petal*.
Eomma kneads kinks out of dough and telephone wire. To invert your body is to hide
the holes in your sleeves, the sloppy stitching, Eomma's hands. I swallow
the warmth and then the words. I drink rivers of smoke. Sometimes,
the only thing separating a body from grief is more grief. Eomma cradles
the landline like an infant. Sometimes, there is quiet. I run and I run.
Eomma asks, *What are you running for?* and today, I have
an answer. A bullet cuts through the window panes and the pigeons
swallow glass. I run towards light, towards smoke.
When disaster blooms, bruise-like, undresses its red body,
Eomma spreads her palms, as if to say, *Welcome.*
As if to say, *We have bent for lesser things*. As if to open.

2004

your name meaning *people's vegetable*

not snowdrop
boughs of ripe jade
full stomach
limbs heavy with bounty

meaning fracture inherited
like something internal
your mouth the sole citizen
of an unspeakable country
your invertebrate of a mouth
pulsing
simultaneous lives of
a people's republic
mouthfuls of steaming bitterness
this allegory for desire
unfulfilled

your name not your name

NEW YEAR

And maybe I won't
go to bed sad any more

than I already do.
Maybe I will find myself

a continent to burrow
into like sleep.
In a soft mountain

somewhere. A wandering city. City
puckered sour and sung sweet.

So sweet
you call it a trick
of the light. Foolish, troubling
light.

Eomma, dear eomma,
are the trees loud where you rest?

You were never unfamiliar.
Because you have burned before.

So human:
like poetry or a child's
laugh or a ruined house.

Spilt like yolk
and embryonic.

So that's the poem.
Vertical descent,
common ancestor,
the spot in the rearview mirror
where your reflection
fails.

Where you vault
the light
and the cicadas, the pale
lining of trees.

I wanted
often. Mutated
from generations of aphids,
their songs and tears
often.

My lightless hair. My grieving,
too. It blooms,

a lonely beginning.

EOMMA'S PANTOUM

Kitchen smoke collecting into fingers, into fists
blooming open. I inherit grief, Eomma's
apron salted with bleach stains,
so many pigeons behind glass. Bodies

blooming open. I inherit grief, Eomma's
way of returning home, nesting, preserving
so many pigeons behind glass. Bodies
can only remember so much. No

way of returning home.
A way of saying, *I*
can only remember so much. No.
I can only say what I mean.

A way of saying
my first language is grief.
I can only say what I mean.
I mean this is all I can say.

I will let it happen. I will swallow the
kitchen smoke, the fingers, fists
still reeling from the punch. There is no grief like an
apron salted with bleach stains.

APPA HAS THIS RECURRING DREAM

in which he is a wandering ghost alone in an auditorium. And although he is a ghost, his footsteps echo, and he is always surrounded by a crowd of moving bodies bathed in fragile light. In his dreams, he is unsure of what he is looking for: a body or a stuttering heartbeat or just an invitation to stay the night, to nurse a warm bowl of soup, anything to distract him from his own ghostliness. Meanwhile, I sleep some nights and wake with dull teeth and a sudden awareness of all that ache concentrated in my mouth. Cool enamel and smooth glass. The way that bone shatters into sharp limbs of snow under pressure. Dream Appa is unable to go to the afterlife, locked inside this cavernous chamber of a heart, and maybe I should have burned more candles. Searched more diligently, clenched my teeth harder. Maybe I coveted too thoughtlessly the way the light falls when it misses heaven, that gleaming star. Appa tells me, dream or not, he is always lonely. After many nights, he tells me he can't pass on because he is waiting in an auditorium, a school auditorium, and it's the night of a big recital, and I'm up there reading a poem. It never matters how late it is, because Appa is always waiting for me to finish my sentence, to catch my breath. It is a lonely haunting, but it is his. He stays so that he can watch me gleam, radioactive under fluorescent light. He does not blink, not even when the people around him mutate into white noise. It is only when I swallow my last word that he shatters into white mirrors, sharp teeth, generations of snowflakes and their silent screams. *Appa, please wait,* I want to say. *Please stay* *a little longer.* But he can't, and we both know this, so instead I stare straight through him: suspended bones, strung tendon, the dull ache of his heart, this ache that never leaves my wordless

mouth.

MANIFESTO FOR THE IMMIGRANT POET

After Theresa Hak Kyung Cha (1951–1982) (aged 31)

1. We are poets, meaning we have something to share.
2. 시 [translation: city] 시 [translation: muse] 시 [translation: poem]
3. We speak with verve, in verse, invert what is invertible and intern what isn't. We are immigrants of an impossible country, that without language or limbs. We raise every word to the sun like a shard of glass, diffracting meaning and extracting light. We are the poet and her poem.
4. Her poem is an attempt at translation. There is no attempt without failure. There is no failure without grief. The poem is a city is a muse is a poem still.
5. 성 [surname] 성 [sex] 성 [holy]
6. We seek the boundaries of definition. In this language, the names that follow us are castles of memory. We collect them like lost coins, loose teeth, losing bets: things worth finding for the sake of joy, however small. We, Korean and American in the same sharp breath. We, the mile-long feast and its stretch of hunger. We, poet, poem.
7. 눈 [eye] 눈 [snow]
8. 새 [bird] 새 [anew]
9. Once, we followed the snow, watched as it blinked. In this language, to ask is to bury. In this language where eyes are less than mirrors, we remember the displaced body is still a body. The immigrant poem is still a poem. We remember this: a bird is a beginning that flutters, a beginning that sings.
10. Just look at the infinite ways in which light can bend.
11. How can I say the world is a cold place?

12. Above the running man is the flying man. Above that, something you cannot imagine.
13. Somewhere, a bird sings.
14. 배 [stomach] 배 [pear] 배 [ship]
15. 묻다 [to ask] 묻다 [to bite] 묻다 [to bury]
16. Our bodies remember displacement in unfinished sentences, a tongue reborn before the roof of a mouth. Blood is denser than water and we know we will sink like the heaviest pears, like bloating stomachs, like a ship nowhere bound—all equal in the bearing of rot. We remember displacement because we have survived it.
17. Here is the body. Dig with the wealth of your hands.
18. We persist. We rise to electric life, occupy every room of our joy. We eat stars and hold grudges. We are made of so much hunger and not enough bite. We are the sum of our parts, or we want to be.
19. Everything we love does not belong to us.
20. Do you remember what was asked?
21. Do you remember how we were buried?
22. 말 [word] 말 [horse]
23. This language is wild, an unruly horse. So we will let it be wild, this untamable language.
24. 시 [ ] 시 [ ] 시 [
25. We are not looking for forgiveness. We are not looking for the good years, the synonyms for survival that fit in the pinch of two fingers. We are looking for a pat of flour on kneaded dough, a sewn patch over skinned knees, another bowl of soup, a body to be sung.
26. We are looking for hunger and it is looking for us.
27. 쓰다 [to write] 쓰다 [to be bitter]

28. The poem is a bitter poem is a poem is a poet is waiting to be found.
29. 시 [neweye] 시 [snowbird] 시 [askaskaskaskbitebury] 시 [biteagain]
30. We will rebuild ourselves, limb by limb, word by word.
31. Something like a country or a crystalline heart or a poem, yes, a poem.

ANTIBODY

I could tell you a lifetime of loss.
Appa's missing butterfly collection
and his waning eyes. Or Eomma's eomma,
her appa, the old home and its old desires.
At the laboratory, I paint
entire lineages radioactive green,
stained fluorescent with protein. I measure
life, entropic tangle, its pulse
and its ache. Particles and their unstable trace.
At home, I swallow wild wormwood, steaming
ginseng, the wet of an unseeing eye.
I track chemicals into the kitchen, dark into
my childhood bedroom. I imagine
Appa's butterflies as they were: hanging
on a wall, wing-first, vision frozen
in colors invisible to us. Creatures nailed

to their impermanence, their living
grace. Always naked and never
warm. And maybe I was too envious
of bright wings against shattered glass,
nuclei saturated with bright beads,
the undeniable glamor of flight. Maybe
you are only ever the way

you exit the world. Because
the light always picks up everything
you try to leave behind. Remember
the winter when deer tracked mud, fresh
with decay, into the foyer? How they nosed
the carpet skittishly, eyes wet
and blind. How we shrugged our shoulders,
as if to free ourselves. Said to the deer,
Come as you are. Stay
a while.

ACKNOWLEDGMENTS

The Adroit Journal: "Murder Hornets"

Beloit Poetry Journal: "Prospect Theory"

The Cincinnati Review: "Sonnet as First Words"

Columbia Journal: "Gloria" and "Sonnet with Kitchen Grease"

Invisible City Literary Journal: "Bildungsroman"

Journal of General Internal Medicine: "Post-Operative Care"

Narrative Magazine: "Aubade in the Aftermath" and "Suite D"

Poetry Magazine: "Respite"

West Branch: "Transit," "Axiom" and "Duplex in San Francisco"

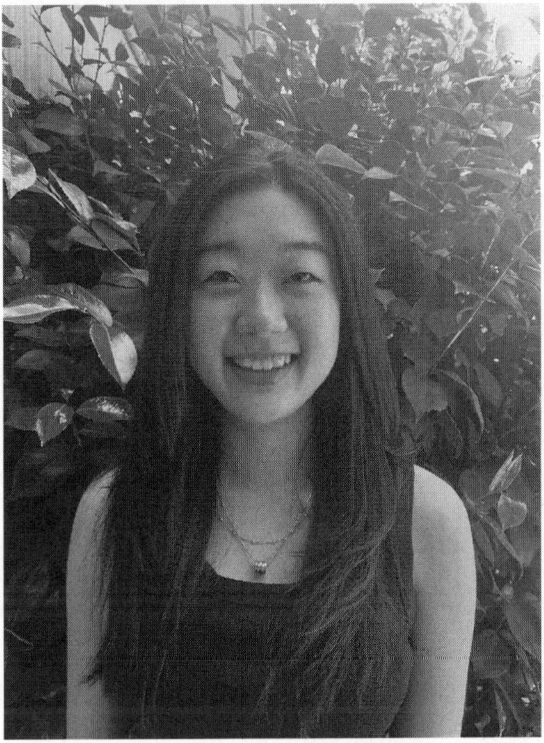

ELANE KIM is a Korean American writer from California. The editor-in-chief of *Gaia Lit*, she is the recipient of the 2024 Roger Conant Hatch Prize for Lyric Poetry, the winner of the 2021 Columbia Journal Winter Poetry Contest, and a Davidson Fellow in Literature. Her writing can be found in *Poetry*, *Narrative Magazine*, *One Teen Story*, and more. She is the author of the chapbook *Postcards* (Bull City Press, 2022) and a student at Harvard College.

RIVER RIVER BOOKS was founded by Amorak Huey and Han VanderHart in March 2022. Inspired by the idea that you cannot step in the same river twice, two poetry editors join together to publish (at least) two exceptional poetry titles a year, as well as the Plainwater Nonfiction Series.

Poetry Catalog

An Eye in Each Square, Lauren Camp, 2023
Bullet Points: A Lyric, Jennifer A Sutherland, 2023
Dear Memphis, Rachel Edelman, 2024
A Geography That Does Not Hurt Us, Carla Sofia Ferreira, 2024
Pastoral, 1994, Joe Wilkins 2025
Your Mother's Bear Gun, Corrie Williamson, 2025
Field Notes, E.G. Cunningham, 2025
Encounters for the Living and the Dead, Jameela F. Dallis, 2025
Antibody, Elane Kim, 2026
House of Myth and Necessity, Jennifer A Sutherland, 2026
Scythe, Elizabeth Sylvia, 2026
Fifty Mothers, Preeti Vangani, 2026
The Visible Field, Zoë Ryder White, 2026
Snails of the Apocalypse, Martha Zweig, 2026
Turn a Girl to Salt, Janet McAdams, 2027
Little Automata of the Deciduous Forest, Mirande Bissell, 2027
Whale Garden, Carolyn Oliver, 2027

Plainwater Nonfiction Series

There Is News Along the Ohio River, Beth Gilstrap, 2026
Backyard Alchemy, J.D. Ho, 2026